compassionate competency:
healing the heart of healthcare

Emelia Sam

ACKNOWLEDGEMENTS

For every patient, student and colleague who has shaped my professional path. To my mentor and friend, Dr. Andrea Bonnick, who has always been a champion for treating patients in a compassionate manner. Thank you for your example.

CONTENTS

Preface   1

Chapter 1   Introduction   5

Chapter 2   Communication   21

Chapter 3   Observation   35

Chapter 4   Mastery   45

Chapter 5   Pausing   55

Chapter 6   Attention   65

Chapter 7   Self-Care   75

Chapter 8   Standards   85

Chapter 9   Integration   89

Chapter 10   Objectivity   95

Chapter 11   Needs   103

Chapter 12   Conclusion   113

PREFACE

For many years, I lived a double life.

Having spent thirteen years on the path of becoming an oral and maxillofacial surgeon, I wouldn't have imagined anything other than satisfaction and pride would await me at the finish line. Though I had occasionally sensed that something was amiss along the way, I simply dismissed it as the pains and sacrifices that I was always told would undoubtedly accompany accomplishment.

But something was unmistakably missing as I settled into my profession. A remote space within my being had been long starved and overlooked in the name of achievement. The structured path I dutifully followed was at the expense of the persistent impulse to write.

For years, I had repeatedly ignored the call. Only in the throes of exaggerated heartache would I permit myself to indulge in the writing of a lovelorn poem. Words never intended for any eyes other than my own.

But the desire to write extended far beyond anguish of the heart. I was a self-help junkie steadily consuming a diet heavy in personal development and spirituality. Along the way, I began publishing my own thoughts on what it meant to evolve, to become a better person, to bring meaning to one's life.

The blogosphere had emerged and using my middle name, I quietly made my contribution as a faceless entity. The double life began.

By day, I held my job as surgeon and professor. By night, or as I like to say, by heart, I wrote short, soulful contemplations, and explored themes of purpose, alignment and compassion.

Needless to say, I saw no overlap in these two areas of my life. I blogged for a few years and published a book entitled *I Haven't Found Myself but I'm Still Looking*. Yet, no one in my professional life knew anything about it.

It wasn't until I read Daniel Pink's *A Whole New Mind* that I began to see the possibility of convergence.

As will be explained in the introductory chapter of this book, empathy is an emerging "conceptual sense" as Pink terms it.[1] As a writer, empathy was a space I frequented. As a doctor, I've always been acutely aware of its deficit in healthcare.

At last, the seemingly incongruent parts of my life finally fit together. The things I never felt permitted to truly explore in my workspace were the things it so desperately needed to move it into the 21st century.

Healthcare needs an overhaul.

However, this isn't the typical makeover we see in various industries; those are the standard attempts at streamlining in an effort to increase productivity and enhance financial payoffs.

This transformation requires a makeover from the inside out. As participants in the healthcare system, we have to take a good look at ourselves.

To solely envision our industry as a "system" is to see it purely as methodology in which we are mere cogs in a wheel. Subjecting the public to automated practices certainly removes the touch of humanity that the word "care" implies.

It is this ongoing challenge that *Compassionate Competency* sets out to address.

Chapter 1
INTRODUCTION

Given that the internet grants access to information on virtually anything, people tend to be more meticulous about their choices. Whether debating upon which restaurant to patronize or which airline offers the best deal, online resources are often considered trusted sources.

Furthermore, rate-based systems and informal rating practices, through the use of real-time social media, sway the decisions of consumers. Healthcare facilities and their practitioners are no exception.

It takes only seconds to find available information on where a practitioner has studied, how many years of experience, and if a history of legal issues exists. And if no information can be found, the individual conducting the search may quickly move to the next choice available.

By doing these crude searches, patients are looking to confirm a level of competence. However, over the years, I noticed an emerging pattern regarding the ways in which patients relate to their chosen doctors. It appeared that expectations exceed the usual parameters by which practitioners have been judged.

I have had numerous conversations in which it felt as if patients were looking for something beyond solely competence.

A Whole New Mind

These conversations reminded me of a book I read years prior, *A Whole New Mind: Why Right-Brainers Will Rule the Future* by Daniel

Pink. It described how our society, dominated by "left-brained thinking" for centuries, has been transitioning to so-called "right brained thinking." In short, the creatives are taking the lead.

As is pointed out in his book, there is no right-brain or left-brain. It works in concert. However, the halves seem to process information differently. The left does so in a sequential, logical order, whereas the right half operates in a simultaneous, big-picture manner.

Another book that comes to mind is *My Stroke of Insight* by neuroanatomist, Jill Bolte-Taylor. She details her experience while having a stroke in the left hemisphere of her brain and her arduous recovery period.[2] Her story is helpful to gain a rudimentary understanding of the differences between how the hemispheres operate. (If you aren't inclined to read another book, you can watch her popular TED talk with the same title.)

Pink effectively uses this left-brain/right-brain paradigm while elucidating on the progression of society. As he outlines, we have progressed through the agrarian age, industrial age, information age and are now in the conceptual age.

Farmers were central in the agrarian age, factory workers in the industrial age, and with the information age/technological period, we have seen the rise of what Pink calls "knowledge workers." These periods have been largely dominated by a logical, "left-brained" focus.

If we look at what has been happening with the emergence of the conceptual age, the creators and empathizers are stepping to the forefront. People are getting more creative with how they present what they present to the world.

For example, you may or may not have noticed the emergence of storytelling. There have always been professional storytellers. However, their skill had not traditionally been considered mainstream in a knowledge worker world.

Now, stories have come to the forefront in how leading brands are marketing and promoting themselves. Social media sites, such as Instagram, are often used to show behind the scenes. They are building relationships with consumers through the stories they are sharing. The sole offering of products and services is no longer enough.

Pink goes on to support his argument pointing out that we live in a world of abundance. Choices are plenty. Information is everywhere. As a result, the things and experiences that people will now demand are the things that can't be replicated.

They want meaning.

This is where the so-called right-brained perspective comes in. Pink outlined what he refers to as the six conceptual senses. (I encourage you to read his book to fully comprehend these concepts.) These are the abilities of individuals who dominate in the current conceptual age.

They are:

Design
Empathy
Story
Symphony
Play
Meaning

While these senses can blend seamlessly, I choose to highlight the one sense that stands out most when it comes to the topic of healthcare – empathy. Surely, there are ways for all of these senses to be incorporated within the industry, but empathy holds particular resonance for me.

Over the last fifteen years, I've seen thousands of patients and have been a patient. I've accompanied loved ones to their appointments, both routine and emergent. I've listened carefully to the accounts of friends and acquaintances who have sought care for a variety of reasons. The spectrum of experience is broad.

I firmly believe that patients have grown tired of being treated in an algorithmic fashion. Computers can do that. And in the age we live in, if patients want to know something, they Google or consult sites such as WebMD.

Though they may be misinformed or wrongly interpret what they find, the initial thought is to go to the computer and not the actual specialist. By the time they come to us, they want more from us than just our knowledge- even if they can't articulate what that *more* is.

This is the "it factor" that exceptional practitioners possess and here is where we venture into the world of emotional intelligence (EQ).

Emotional Intelligence

As defined by Oxford dictionary, emotional intelligence is

"the capacity to be aware of, control, and express one's emotions, and to handle

interpersonal relationships judiciously and empathetically."

(Sounds like the key to good bedside/chairside manner, no?)

Mayer, Salovey, and Caruso developed the emotional intelligence test (MSCEIT) in 1990 although the concept or similar terms had been used in prior research. However, in 1995, Daniel Goleman wrote the groundbreaking book, *Emotional Intelligence*, based off of the researchers' findings.

His stance is that of EQ being equal to if not more important than IQ for personal and professional success.[3] If we relate this to the simplistic left brain/right-brain model, then IQ would be considered left as EQ would be considered right.

Why is this important? Over the last few decades, we have seen how technology has exploded. In many areas, computers have replaced humans. IQ has been and continues to be replicated.

It is EQ that sets us apart. When is the last time you were frustrated interacting with some form of automation and wanted nothing more than a human being who understood what you required?

In addition, unlike IQ, emotional intelligence is something that can be nurtured. There are multiple school-based programs teaching techniques to children in order to produce well-adjusted adults.

But what about the rest of us? How can we cultivate these characteristics within ourselves? Certainly, these skills could be useful personally and professionally.

Mindfulness

In comes the current buzzword, mindfulness. We see it being mentioned not only in pop culture, but in corporate culture. It is no longer exclusively associated with the yoga-loving, organic eating, tree-hugging individual. (By the way, there's nothing wrong with that if you fit the description.)

The practice of mindfulness has made its way into bedrooms and boardrooms. Over the years it has become increasingly integrated into healthcare.

What is mindfulness? According to Jon Kabat-Zinn, the man who popularized the practice in the West, mindfulness is,

"to purposefully pay attention in a sustained and non-judgmental way to what is going on in your body, your mind, and the world around you."

In 1979, Jon Kabat-Zinn created an eight-week course called Mindfulness Based Stress Reduction (MBSR) in the Stress Reduction Clinic at the University of Massachusetts Medical School. The course was aimed at patients with chronic pain.

The popularity of MBSR has grown since the 90s and highly certified teachers offer the course worldwide. However, the student demographics have extended far beyond the chronic pain population. It is available to anyone wanting to reduce stress.

There are even specific courses aimed at practitioners in healthcare professions.

In addition, there have been several medical schools and a few dental schools that have implemented these programs as electives. The learned skills mitigate the stresses of these highly competitive environments and will continue to aid these individuals once they enter their professional lives.

Relevance

Emotional intelligence allows us to be more effective practitioners as we can accurately sense our patients' needs beyond textbook treatment. It allows for greater overall professionalism. Equally important, it promotes personal well-being which can only enhance the aforementioned benefits.

In addition, for those of us who act in a teaching capacity, it gives us insight on student perspectives so we can teach more effectively. And, by example, we pass on life-changing skills to our pupils.

We have been educated and educate others to be clinically competent. But this is not enough for the direction that healthcare is headed.

The academic aspect and the logistics of healthcare are continually addressed and revised. However, the emotional aspects of extending and receiving care have not been a primary focus. As a result, we have far too many disgruntled patients and fatigued and/or ineffective practitioners.

Compassion has been the missing piece and this is how we cultivate it. We start with ourselves and extend it outwardly.

Compassionate Competency attempts to combine "right-brained sensibilities" with the tenets of emotional intelligence and practices of mindfulness.

Using compassion as a mnemonic, this work highlights skills, practices, and ideals embodied by 21st century practitioners and educators of those practitioners.

Communication

Observation

Mastery

Pausing

Attention

Self-Care

Standards

Integration

Objectivity

Needs

Chapter 2
COMMUNICATION

Communication forms the basis of every relationship. Whether parent-child, educator-student, or practitioner-patient, the ways in which we communicate define the nature of the interactions. It also sets the tone for whatever follows those exchanges.

Traditionally, caregivers (especially doctors) have approached patients in a parental manner. There was little to suggest in formal education that we should do otherwise.

Most curricula focused on imparting didactic and clinical information without regard to the caregiver-patient dynamic. Fortunately, over the years we are seeing more and more emphasis on effective communication being integrated into studies.

The "I know more than you, so do what I say" approach may have seemed more acceptable when information was exclusive. In today's culture, that is no longer the case.

Access Granted

Unless a patient had formal training or an inquisitive disposition, there wouldn't be, or perhaps more accurately, *couldn't* be engaged discourse. Now, gone are the days of dispensing information in the tradition of one-way conversations.

Given the climate of infinite access to information, more patients are finding their voices. Many are interested in being an active participant in their healthcare rather than a passive recipient. They show up armed with information and are more apt to ask questions.

However, the independent research isn't always accurate due to the abundance of unverified sources. Anyone with an opinion can start a blog and create a following. Unfortunately, individuals won't always be able to discern fact from fiction and may only be relying upon popularity as an indication of expertise.

Whether today's patient is informed or misinformed, the nature of conventional interactions continues to transform. As healthcare practitioners, we must be willing to have conversations we never would have had even ten years ago.

While some may consider this bothersome, the upside is that it keeps us on our toes. If new information is available, we have to be able to expand on it should a patient bring it up, or debunk it as necessary.

While independent "Googling" and "YouTubing" will never match the structured roads of certification and licensure, we must be sure not to dismiss patients in their earnest efforts. This new dynamic requires us to become allies as opposed to daunting authorities. There's no place for intimidation if we are truly interested in best outcomes for our patients.

Listen Up

Author and physician, Dr. Danielle Ofri, writes and speaks on various topics within the realm of medicine. Her book, *What Patients Say, What Doctors Hear*, is an extensive exploration of communication between physicians and patients.

One point that resonated deeply is something I see as rampant in healthcare environments. (Actually, it's rampant in all environments.) Our inability or unwillingness to listen is a huge disservice to those we supposedly serve.

How often do we cut short the telling of a patient's narrative? How often do we rush them to get to the point? How often are we concerned or annoyed at what we perceive as rambling? How many cues do we miss in our haste?

In jumping from patient to patient or task to task, we compromise effective communication in the name of efficiency. Consequently, we're not necessarily helping the process of healing; we are managing.

Listening is a vital skill and, fortunately, one that can be cultivated. As mentioned in Ofri's book, Dr. Daniel Boudreau, from the McGill Centre for Medical Education, developed a course in "attentive listening."[4]

Medical students were taken through exercises which included: discerning amongst identical classical pieces played by three different pianists, noting differences in a patient's tone pre- and post-depression, and paying attention to the specific words patients chose when sharing their narratives.

In essence, the course was designed to help students not only in hearing what was said, but to take note of subtleties and "hear" between the lines.

To see this aspect of healthcare being addressed in a formal manner is quite encouraging. However, many of us who have long since graduated from our respective programs haven't received this type of training. Perhaps we'll see more of it incorporated into continuing education opportunities. We can all stand to sharpen our communication skills.

Back to the Basics

Not everyone is blessed with charisma. That is a quality that cannot be taught. However, all of us can improve our interactions by paying attention to the basics.

By being in an academic environment, I often observe some very awkward exchanges as students start to navigate clinical environments. Unfortunately, there are some of the same behaviors I've witnessed (or experienced as a patient) from seasoned practitioners.

1. A simple introduction goes a long way.

It's not uncommon for a nervous student or a rushed practitioner to forget their manners. Jumping straight to patient concerns, especially if you are new to the patient, can make for an uncomfortable situation. An introduction and/or an exchange of pleasantries takes a few seconds and most people react favorably to an initial warm-up.

2. Make eye contact.

This is such a simple but crucial act. Taking notes is important but in between jotting points down or typing them out, make sure to reorient yourself to the person in front of you.

Eye contact indicates you are paying attention and fosters a certain level of trust. Otherwise, a patient that feels unheard and unseen will likely become frustrated which in turn may frustrate you.

3. Don't interrupt.

It's highly unlikely that a patient will use up a tremendous amount of time describing their issues. We're often impatient and want to eliminate what we believe to be extraneous information.

However, relevant matters may reveal themselves in a slightly longer narrative. Once again, this goes to making the patient feel heard. Remember, this is not a case you are trying to solve. It's a person you're aiming to help.

4. Meet at eye level.

You never want to talk down to your patients, figuratively or literally. Standing over a patient isn't necessary unless one is performing an examination or procedure.

It may seem like a little thing, but body language, including the way you position yourself, sets a tone. There are theories that your posture and positioning can influence your behavior subconsciously and consequently, that of those around you.

When we interact with a patient who is positioned at an inferior level, what is the underlying message? As stated earlier, the parental approach is outdated and patients need not be made to feel as though they hold no power.

5. Speak plainly.

Sharing accurate information is of the utmost importance. Using clinical terms only becomes a problem when not explained in layman's language. I can't count the number of times I've heard practitioners using formal language, while also missing the mystified look on the faces of their patients. (See #2)

6. Invite questions.

One-way conversations have no place in today's healthcare environment. If we are truly interested in serving the people who come to us, we must make space for them to participate.

Effective communicators aren't only interested in delivering a message. They want to make sure that message is heard and correctly understood. This is one of the primary aims of a compassionately competent practitioner.

The Core Message

Whatever your particular role may be when dealing with patients, the essential art of communication cannot be overlooked. The following words sum things up nicely with great insight and a pinch of humor.

> *"The biggest take-home message for me, after wading through the research and interviewing people on all sides of the issue, is that both doctors and patients need to give communication its just due. Rather than seeing the conversation between doctor and patient as the utilitarian humdrum of a visit, the conversation should be viewed as the single most important tool of medical care. It*

should be given the deference and attention that we lavish upon the swankiest of medical technologies.

If you consider the amount of information that can be gleaned from a doctor-patient conversation, the diagnoses that can be made, the analyses that can be elaborated, the treatments that can be rendered, the human connections that can be cultivated— the simple conversation is, in fact, a highly sophisticated technology. It's far more intricate, powerful, and flexible than most of our other medical technologies, which generally do only one thing in only one way. Plus, conversation is way cheaper and it doesn't decimate your sex drive or make you puke."

~ Danielle Ofri, MD, PhD
What Patients Say, What Doctors Hear

Enough said.

Chapter 3
OBSERVATION

As healthcare providers, our powers of observation are crucial. We are trained to see what patients, themselves, may miss. And, what we fail to see can be, at worst, fatal.

It is often assumed that experience will train the eyes of practitioners; that over the years, observation skills will undoubtedly improve. While this is so, it seems a rather passive way to develop such an important skill.

Early on in my teaching career, I used to marvel at how new students could miss what I thought to be glaringly obvious. In the span of a few years, I had distanced myself from the memory of my own untrained eye.

I had forgotten that I had to build my catalogue of observations. With each patient encounter, I would store away pertinent information. After enough encounters, I would then be able to identify specific traits.

In clinical situations, I would see a condition and search my database (experiential and textbook) to find a corresponding representation. It was a rather robotic approach, similar to using facial recognition software.

Though effective, this matching strategy doesn't allow for detection of subtleties. It allows for black and white identification while missing the grays.

Traditionally, the emphasis has been on how to treat what is observed. It hasn't necessarily focused upon teaching *how* to observe. Thankfully, other methods are now being employed to develop a critical eye.

The Art of Observation

The world of technology has introduced increasingly sophisticated diagnostic aids. Unfortunately, as they have emerged, the primary tools of communication and observation have taken a backseat.

Patients can often feel that their interactions with healthcare workers only serve to get the preliminaries out of the way. From their perspective, it may seem that they are being treated according to a predetermined checklist; only lab results and radiology studies appear to matter. Sadly, this happens far too often.

Due to modern conveniences, there is less focus on the skills that ultimately create connection. Instead of working in concert, technology is often placed ahead of humanity.

It is absolutely true that these tests can often detect what the human eye cannot. However, that should not mean we disregard our basic abilities and associated intuitive skills. Indeed, we may be missing out on invaluable wisdom. How can we begin to access this space within ourselves?

In the introductory chapter, I touched on "right-brain sensibilities" as described in *A Whole New Mind.* While clinical examination and assessment seemingly fall under the category of "left-brained," there is much to be learned from our creative counterparts.

Once again, the interplay of art and science may prove to be a saving grace. The last chapter mentioned an innovative course that helped medical students to improve their listening skills.

Since 2005, Harvard Medical School has offered the elective course, *Training the Eye.* It was started by Dr. Joel Katz and Dr. Shahram Khoshbin and is available to medical students at all levels. The course aims to enhance the "visual literacy" of course participants.[5,6]

During the ten-week curriculum, students commit to visits to the Boston Museum of Fine

Arts, drawing instruction, didactics and patient rounds. The idea is to develop skills that can be transferred to clinical environments. The combination of these activities has proven to be highly beneficial.

By the end of the course, students have been shown to be more observant with an increased ability to express those observations as compared to students who did not participate. They also tend to provide more evidence for their interpretations of clinical findings. In addition, they develop awareness with respect to their underlying biases and judgments making for more objective assessments.

This reminds me of an interview I recently heard with Dr. Terry Wahls, clinical professor of medicine at the University of Iowa. Prior to her medical training, she received a bachelor's degree in fine arts.

In recalling her years in med school, she stated,

"It was very clear, when we entered the clinical world, I had a different point of view. I was much more interested in the patient narrative and I had (from my point of view) a better sense of observation, the details on the physical exam, the subtleties. Visual orientation was so much stronger for me than my colleagues."[7]

Dr. Terry Wahls
Good Life Project Podcast

Dr. Shahram shared that through alumni, this course has spread to other institutions and that the list keeps growing. They have also instructed others in advanced educational techniques under the arts and humanities initiative at Harvard Medical School.

All in all, the integration of art only helps to enhance our skillsets. The study of art allows us to fine tune our senses in such a way that traditional clinical study does not address.

Technology can gather and provide the type of information that the world of "knowledge workers" has always sought. However, today's healthcare worker must seek to reach beyond that.

This isn't just about developing a more critical eye. By taking the time to tap into and use our human skills, we create something far more valuable. Ultimately, we create the connections that technology cannot.

Chapter 4
MASTERY

Imagine an eight-year-old child dressed up as a physician for Halloween. Chances are that you are picturing an oversized costume consisting of the well-known symbols associated with the profession:

White coat
Stethoscope
Old-school headlamp
Black bag

Even though the last two items are somewhat outdated, they speak to how engrained cultural stereotypes are. (Note: Housecalls are making a comeback so we may see more of those doctors' bags.) Picture a nurse's costume, and the all-white outfit complete with stockings and a cap comes to mind. I don't remember seeing either representation in person within my lifetime, yet the images are firmly planted.

Though much has changed and traditional wear has been widely replaced with more informal scrubs, some of the visual cues persist. For example, hospital and clinic personnel often wear white coats. (As an aside, I haven't worn a white coat in years. Perhaps, a quietly rebellious act on my part.)

The point is that we often identify professionals largely by their appearance. The assumption is that the wearer of the "costume" holds specialized knowledge and has been deemed competent. In a healthcare setting, that white coat is supposed to signify members of health professions.

What the attire cannot speak to is the character of the individual. All the tests may have been passed and all the licenses obtained; yet, he or she may be highly arrogant, socially inept, or possess any other disastrous combination of undesirable characteristics. Just because someone has acquired professional status doesn't mean they exhibit professionalism.

The Consummate Professional

The Merriam-Webster dictionary defines professionalism as "the conduct, aims, or qualities that characterize or mark a profession or a professional person."

The majority of people would probably agree upon this definition. However, I find it peculiar that most of the presentations I have seen on professionalism, almost always start with attire. It's almost as if at least "looking the part" takes importance over embodying it. After all, there are those who still take offense to the concept of "casual Fridays."

More than likely, it is because addressing the abstract nature of character proves difficult whereas definitive checklists for clothing are easily provided. Nonetheless, we know that professionalism goes well beyond appearance to include such things as: demeanor, ethical behavior, accountability, reliability and, of course, competence.

What is it that shapes these other qualities? I strongly believe the determinant is self-mastery.

Know Thyself

As described by Daniel Goleman, self-mastery is the result of self-awareness combined with self-regulation.[8] In the book, *The Brain and Emotional Intelligence: New Insights*, Goleman describes neurological findings regarding the interaction between the prefrontal cortex and the amygdala.

In case you need a refresher, the amygdala is the emotional center. It is the part of the brain that is on high alert looking out for threats. Unfortunately, it tends to be overly reactive.

The pre-frontal cortex is the site for rationale. It is the area that inhibits much (but not all!) of our inappropriate behavior. The interplay of these two areas determines the degree of self-control one exhibits. It all depends on who is winning the tug-of-war.

The good news is that one can learn to counter the impulse to over-react. Goleman suggests various methods:

1. Cognitive intervention

Attention is key. Noticing that the emotional state has taken over is the first step. Your better half, so to speak, can step in and rationalize. In other words, you talk yourself off the ledge.

2. Empathy

If involved in an interaction with another, you may choose to pretend you are in their shoes.

Re-evaluate the situation from their perspective. This may quell your emotional state.

3. Biological approach

Relaxation methods, including meditation, have physiological effects. They activate the parasympathetic nervous system which is in opposition to an alarmed state. However, Goleman cautions that this is only effective for the individual who is practiced in their chosen method.

Having mastery over oneself means everything if one is to exhibit professionalism. It is what allows a sense of accountability. It is what keeps an individual from being subject to random external influences.

Mastery places you in the driver's seat. You can witness your own emotional states, identify and modify as necessary. It creates the space for stronger decision-making and ethical behavior. It dictates overall demeanor and promotes personal well-being.

Without question, greater self-awareness allows for improved relationships with patients. Being attuned to personal states allows one to more accurately sense that of others. Consequently, it can change the entire dynamic.

Mastery is what separates the individual who looks and acts the part of a professional from those fully embodying professionalism. And the best part about cultivating mastery is that is only requires your willingness.

Chapter 5
PAUSING

The power of the pause can never be underestimated. No matter how busy one may claim to be, there is always room for this one simple practice. Furthermore, it is a gift available to each of us if we are aware enough to choose it.

Be it thirty seconds or thirty minutes, a conscious break in activity has the potential to be highly restorative. We've all felt the rejuvenation of a brief walk outside or a quick stretch after sitting in front of a computer screen.

I believe that the inherent strength of pausing doesn't come from the break itself, but what potentially can happen in the break. I share the following story to illustrate.

Sometime ago, I heard about the University of Virginia Medical Center trauma team. As you can imagine or may have experienced, being in an emergency environment means being repeatedly presented with dire situations.

It is no wonder that over time, any team may become desensitized to the passing of patients. That is not to say they become indifferent to death, but there is a hardening or distancing, a protective response that many will experience.

But in this particular emergency room, one nurse, made a conscious decision to act differently. After the passing of a patient, Jonathan Bartels simply paused.[9]

He stopped to take in the moment.

This was highly uncharacteristic behavior. In a

situation that often functions as a well-oiled machine, moving efficiently onto the next matter, he interrupted the routine.

He continued this practice, invited others to join and the behavior spread to his colleagues. As a collective, it is now a part of their practice to pause after every death. The "business as usual" paradigm has been replaced.

The behavior spread beyond the walls of emergency to other departments and has even gone on to influence other hospitals. Apparently, compassion is contagious.

In his own words, Bartels reflects on the impact:

> *"Healthcare has made phenomenal advances in scientific and technological care of people across the world. In the process of promoting professionalism and embracing the technological advances, I found that we may have lost our connection with 'the heart of healthcare.' Compassion for oneself and compassion for the person we care for can be*

lost in the process of our technological caring.

In 2008 I implemented the Pause in a busy level 1 trauma center to promote healing for the caregiver team, the family and the patient after a death. This practice has changed the way death is approached both nationally and internationally. It has brought the heart back to an entity that was losing its pulse."

~*Jonathan Bartels, RN*

The trauma response scenario is one that many of us will never experience. However, the takeaway is an important one because it illustrates one resounding lesson.

The Importance of the Pause

The pause allows you to get in touch with your basic humanity.

Why is this important? Because this is the space where empathy and compassion live.
In this worst-case scenario of dealing with a death, the ensuing dynamics are changed. Perhaps, the body is handled more reverently. Maybe, the physician approaches the family of the deceased with palpable care and concern.

It is less likely that cold, sterile interactions will take place. With a pause, everything shifts.

In a space where detachment is often the norm (perhaps expected and sometimes even encouraged) something much more human is allowed to take over.

We are not automatons. However, in our professional environments we often act as such. We follow the protocols, finish the tasks, and repeat the behaviors until the day is done.

By implementing a pause, one is allowed a chance to reconnect which is not only an appropriate show of respect in delicate situations, but also an act of self-compassion.

The go-go-go mentality leaves little space to be kind to oneself. And in that state we are less likely to be observant, patient, or kind to those we encounter.

In the realm of healthcare, the people with whom we deal are often in a position bearing some degree of vulnerability. We cannot afford to exacerbate the problems of those we serve with our own unattended issues. We must repeatedly connect with our humanity in order to extend it.

Implementation

Reflect on how you may be able to give yourself breathing space at regular intervals. Perhaps every two hours or five minutes between patients. Whatever works for your particular schedule. Set alarms if need be.

Your pause could be a quick walk, a standard stretch, a few minutes of music, a mini-meditation, or absolutely nothing. There are no rules and it need not be elaborate.

The nature of our work can be very depleting. Your goal here is reconnection and revitalization. Burnout is a very real concern in this industry. Chapter 7 will cover self-care in general, but this speaks to a practice you can implement throughout the day.

To effectively and comprehensively help our patients, we must attend to our own mental states. Optimal care comes from optimized caregivers. Simply pausing grants us the opportunity to offer our best by first being at our best.

Chapter 6
ATTENTION

In a world of mounting distraction, attention feels like a dying art form. While we benefit greatly from technological advances, we must keep in mind the ways our culture is subsequently shaped by that which we have created and continue to create.

In his book *The Shallows: What the Internet is Doing to Our Brains*, Nicholas Carr explores how use of the internet changes us at the neurological level. Countless research supports the idea that much of our online interactions encourage "cursory reading, hurried and distracted thinking, and superficial learning."[10]

We're sifting through large amounts of information in minimal amounts of time. We're deciding which links to click and which to ignore. Meanwhile, we're receiving hits of dopamine from audible pings signaling new email in our inboxes or any other number of notifications.

Throw in offline concerns such as household tasks, paying bills, or any miscellaneous item on the day's to-do list, and cognitive chaos ensues.

The Myth of Multitasking

Multitasking once referred to the capabilities of computers. Over time, it has come to be applied to humans and many of us proudly claim the badge of "multi-tasker."

Perhaps that has more to do with our culture of busy-ness than our actual ability. Most evidence points to the fact that we are inefficient when it comes to our brains processing simultaneous tasks that each requires significant cognitive effort. Only when tasks are non-competitive can we perform them at the same time.

Whenever we switch from one mode to another, there is a delay in which we disengage from one activity, retrieve the "rules" for the next activity, then execute said activity. There is no parallel processing or instantaneous jump from one to the other.[11]

We tend to process serially. That is true even for the millennial you witness texting on a phone, listening to music, while doing homework on a laptop. We may think their brains are equipped to handle such activity, but efficiency decreases for them as well.

Though our brains may function differently in response to these new cultural habits, that does not mean all of those changes are beneficial. The appearance of new cognitive processes may be at the expense of others.

As stated in the previous chapter, we are not automatons. We must be able to release this harmful notion that we can act as such- especially in the realm of healthcare. We can't afford to be distracted when an individual's well-being is in our hands.

When interacting with a patient, focus must be placed upon that individual. One may be making notes while listening to what is being said seeing as how those are complementary processes. Checking text messages, while taking a health history, is not complementary. These activities compete for attention and focus is shattered.

Proponents of mindfulness would call for an individual to "be in the moment." As new age as that may sound to some, it is an important characteristic to cultivate. Presence makes for exceptional practitioners.

The Power of Presence

Once divorced from the multitasking narrative, healthcare providers become far more valuable in the roles they play professionally and personally.

First, being focused on the task at hand decreases the likelihood of errors. We are human which means mistakes will be made. We cannot eliminate them but we can certainly minimize the occurrence.

Recent studies have claimed that medical errors may be the third leading cause of death in the United States.[12] Moreover, it has been suggested that the estimated number of almost 250,000 individuals per year may be low due to underreporting.

There are undoubtedly several measures that could be taken to avoid a multitude of errors. Indeed, these may include technology or other innovations. However, cultivating a more attentive culture is something immediately available to all.

The second benefit of increased attention is patient connection, literally and figuratively. I was recently listening to an interview with palliative care physician, BJ Miller. As a result of an accident during his sophomore year at college, Dr. Miller had both legs amputated below the knee as well as his left forearm.

He commented that when he first meets a patient, they are assured that he has been in their shoes. Because of his appearance, there is an instant rapport.[13]

The classic clinical interaction can be uncomfortable for many patients. Traditionally, it has not fostered an atmosphere of equality or empathy and unless a practitioner has excellent bedside or chairside manner, true connection is often overlooked.

When Dr. Miller enters the room, the distance between patient and physician disappears because they know he has been on the receiving end of care.

When most of us encounter a patient for the first time, the connection must be established. It is when we pay undivided attention to a patient, that rapport is built. This is the human touch we crave whether we are able to articulate it or not. The connection may even show itself in the most miraculous of ways.

It has been shown that when patients feel connected to their doctors, there is a syncing up in their physiology. Their heart rates tended to match. This phenomenon is known as entrainment.[8]

How remarkable that we are able to witness (and measure) connection; we have physical representation of what we sense about the non-physical. Clinging to the myth of proficient multitasking prevents this type of bridging between patient and provider.

The third benefit of cultivating attention is not only in being able to extend it to patients, but to be able to turn it inward. When we're routinely distracted, not only are we removed from those we serve, but also we become detached from one's own sense of self.

In the previous chapter, the importance of pausing was highlighted. In the following chapter, we delve into the extended conversation of self-care.

Chapter 7
SELF-CARE

"Self-care is the intentional act of doing something to benefit your emotional, physical, and mental well-being." ~RAINN.org

The concept of self-care has been steadily increasing its pervasiveness in culture over the years. We've seen the emergence of whole industries, primarily the wellness and spa industry, overtly centered upon it. However, pampering isn't the only representation of what self-care looks like for varied populations.

The term "work-life balance" has grown in popularity as quality of life has become an increasing concern for people. This echoes Daniel Pink's assertion that people are looking for meaning and depth concerning how their lives are lived. .

Hard work has been a long-admired virtue, but for many individuals the relentless pace of the rat-race is no longer acceptable at the expense of personal well-being. The concept of working one's self into the ground mercilessly is now constantly being questioned.

This is especially important with the healthcare industry. How do we give appropriate care if we aren't caring for ourselves? What comes to mind is the overused but common example of securing one's own oxygen mask before helping others. And yet, well-being is consistently sacrificed in the world of healthcare.

Once dismissed as pop psychology, burnout has become increasingly recognized as a serious issue over the last four decades. While this is true throughout numerous industries, studies show that healthcare professionals are particularly susceptible.

The reasons for burnout may vary: heavy patient loads, limited resources, workplace dynamics, etc. However, the resultant combination of exhaustion, detachment, and a decreased sense of personal accomplishment does not bode well for caregivers or for the recipients of their care.

In one study performed by the American Medical Association and Mayo Clinic, over 6000 physicians were surveyed.[14] The first part of the study in 2011 reported that 45% of them met the criteria for burnout. Just three years later, in 2014, that number had increased to 54.4%. In other surveys conducted across healthcare workers in general, up to 60% report signs of burnout.

The causes of burnout are numerous and so must be the ways in which it is addressed. Not only is significant restructuring in how care is delivered necessary in many spaces, individuals may have to seriously evaluate if they are a good match to the profession at all. Not everyone is built for the sometimes delicate interactions with patients whether in clinical or administrative settings.

Assuming that an individual is suited to their specific profession, then self-care becomes an essential approach to warding off the potential for burnout.

The need for attention to the wellness of healthcare practitioners has not gone unnoticed. As mentioned earlier, The Center for Mindfulness, founded by Jon Kabat-Zinn, offers trainings and retreats specifically aimed at healthcare professionals.

The journey of endodontist, Dr. Christina Pastan, is a wonderful example of the importance of self-care and how it can be integrated into professional spaces. A few years into private practice, stress was starting to take its toll. As a result, she started on a path that would lead her on a journey involving meditation and yoga.

Years later, she would have an opportunity to share her experiential knowledge with a dental resident who was having a panic attack. In the midst of her pupil's crisis, Dr. Pastan was able to teach her a breathing exercise which brought immense relief.

The student would later express profound appreciation for the new life skill she had acquired and Dr. Pastan began to see where she had much more to contribute beyond her dental expertise. She subsequently completed a certification program in yoga instruction through the Kripalu Center for Yoga and Health with the intention of teaching it to students.

In the fall of 2015, she was appointed as the Director of Mind-Body Wellness at Tufts University School of Dental Medicine in Boston, Massachusetts. Dr. Pastan currently offers yoga classes in the school and has collaborated with colleagues to formally incorporate wellness into the student curriculum.

Though introduced as a measure to counter student stresses, the message of self-care extends beyond the student body. Imagine the shift if we were to formally incorporate wellness measures into all of our professional and educational spaces.

Instead of individuals having to seek information and acquire tools on their own, well-being would already be an integrated part of our professions. Knowing the inherent challenges of being in our respective fields, there should be a preventative and supportive approach to addressing the issues.

The under-recognized topic of burnout and its sequelae would no longer be an afterthought. The challenges could be addressed in real-time for students and professionals.

Even without formal introduction or attendance at specifically designed events or programs, the opportunities for personal wellness are endless. What can you regularly do for yourself that will have a cumulative effect on your own well-being?

1. Get physical – walking, hiking, yoga…
2. Ensure adequate sleep.
3. Stay hydrated.
4. Eat nutritiously.
5. Practice meditation.
6. Start gardening.
7. Cook a gourmet meal.
8. Play an instrument.
9. Listen to music.
10. Take up pottery.
11. Learn a foreign language.
12. Read leisurely.
13. Join a book club.
14. Pamper yourself.
15. Write in a journal.
16. Get offline.
17. Bask in solitude.
18. Book a retreat.
19. Get some sun.
20. Hire help for tasks you no longer wish to do.
21. Find a support group.

Self-care takes many forms. It's just a matter of finding what resonates with you. Keeping yourself replenished not only enhances your well-being, It will enhance the quality of care you deliver.

Chapter 8
STANDARDS

The brevity of this chapter is in no way a commentary on its level of importance. The discussion of empathy, compassion and well-being are not routinely discussed in this context and thus require elaboration.

When it comes to standards, the realm of healthcare is more than familiar with the concept. We are extremely comfortable with creating rules and regulations to govern our practices. It's easier to address behavior that can be seen and evaluated as opposed to character, which cannot.

All that being said, forward thinking providers aiming to revise the system have no intention of abandoning the traditional measures and requirements for competence. We want to amend, not dismantle.

It goes without saying that members of the healthcare community must have appropriate training and testing. The lives of others are at stake and there should be no room to allow individuals of questionable capability.

Beyond the rigors of accredited programs, most healthcare workers have to go through some type of certification and/or licensure process. This ensures another level of verification.

Even when an individual has met such qualifications, they are still subject to the scrutiny of their peers. Our professional organizations define the acceptable parameters within which we work in our respective fields. They exist to advocate for the individual but also seek to protect the integrity of a particular occupation.

When it comes to the exploration of standards, it is more than apparent that we build layer upon layer upon layer. We want to ensure such things as sound judgment, clinical skill, and legal compliance. We want to uniformly address concerns such as safety measures and so on.

While healthcare continues to build upon this stratified structure, it must not overlook deficiencies that can't be accredited, tested, or certified.

Standards are important because they speak to the question of what you can and should do. The rest of the Compassionate Competency elements address the question of who you are and consequently *how* you do what the standards stipulate.

Chapter 9
INTEGRATION

The integrity of the healthcare system is greatly compromised. This is not in reference to the morality of the industry. By integrity, I mean wholeness. Its fragmented nature doesn't lend itself to producing the best possible outcomes.

In 1999, the Institute of Medicine (IOM) published *To Err is Human: Building a Better Health System.* The report unflinchingly revealed multiple inadequacies within healthcare that tragically compromised thousands of patients yearly.[15]

In an effort to decrease the chances of human error and promote a "culture of safety" multiple recommendations were made. Amongst them was the example of a collaborative education effort to improve the relations between nurses and physicians; the idea being that improved communications and team-building could optimize circumstances.

The concept of an interdisciplinary approach had been explored for decades. However, there had not been a widespread effort to adopt such practices. After the IOM report, the topic was revisited.

Currently, the terms interprofessional education (IPE) and interprofessional collaborative practice are commonly used. The addition of IPE programs to medical school curricula is steadily increasing.

As defined by the World Health Organization (WHO), IPE

"occurs when students from two or more professions learn about, from and with each

other to enable effective collaboration and improve health outcomes."

"Interprofessional collaborative practice occurs when multiple health workers from different professional backgrounds provide comprehensive health services by working with patients, their families, carers (caregivers), and communities to deliver the highest quality of care across settings."[16]

The need for interprofessional education became highly apparent to me during my days in residency. It was clear that many of the people I worked with, outside of my department, had no idea what my specialty entailed.

On more than one occasion my qualifications and aptitude were questioned by misinformed residents, nurses and attending physicians. It was clear they had a stereoptypical view of dentistry and knew far, far less about my realm of oral and maxillofacial surgery.

On one occasion, a resident asked another individual as if I wasn't in the room, "Are they allowed to write prescriptions?" On another occasion, a nurse delayed fulfilling the orders I had written for an admitted patient on the floor, while I was rotating through a different department.

As irritated as I may have occasionally been, I came to realize that some healthcare workers were no more informed than the lay person about matters outside of their expertise.

To improve the quality of care provided to patients, it is imperative we learn to work in a collaborative manner. We must be educated and ready to expand our very limited definitions of "colleague."

Working from within our silos is no longer acceptable and IPE works to dissolve these boundaries. In order to deliver safe and comprehensive care, it is critical that we integrate our efforts.

Chapter 10
OBJECTIVITY

I share the following experience as an example. Please note, I make no reference to time or place and have changed the name so as to protect patient privacy.

Mr. Smith was man in his sixties who had suffered a major stroke years earlier. Because of his profound impairment, he was confined to a wheelchair. He was unable to communicate through words and could only manage to make loud, protracted moaning-like sounds.

The usual facial expressions were absent due to his paralysis. Yet, there was sadness in his eyes, an exhaustion that was visible to those who were observant. He had little reaction to my greeting of him. In retrospect, I assume he had little expectation.

Mr. Smith, had been bounced from facility to facility, clinic to clinic. He was in pain, of which the source had been recently determined. His caretaker son, who was visibly frustrated, accompanied him to our consultation.

The son recounted the story of his father being repeatedly ignored. Because he was unable to speak, people assumed he was mentally challenged and didn't have the capacity to comprehend. Too many people had spoken around him as if he wasn't there and only addressed the son.

Because there were treatment areas in which the son could not enter, his father unable to advocate for himself, was "set aside" more than once. This more than explained the palpable apathy surrounding Mr. Smith.

A quick examination revealed that despite his larger physical limitations, Mr. Smith was able to open his mouth without issue. He was able to comply with instructions. There was nothing impeding treatment. I assured him (and his son) we would complete his procedure on his subsequent visit. They both appeared reinvigorated by the promise.

On the day of his procedure, treatment was efficiently delivered by a fellow colleague and the gratitude shown by Mr. Smith was immeasurable.

His face was completely lit up and though his attempts to smile were hindered by his physical limitations, his intention was abundantly clear. His "thank you's" were emphatic moans.

His son pulled me aside to express his thanks and proceeded to tell me more about his father. He shared that Mr. Smith had been an accountant prior to the stroke. He referred to him as "brilliant with numbers" and how devastating his stroke had been. His pride in his father was evident.

I am more than certain that though the son was pleased his father was helped with his dental condition, he was more grateful for the fact his father had been *seen*.

Where Bias Lives

This story illustrates many of the principles already covered. It definitely involved communication, observation and attention. However, I choose to highlight objectivity.

In daily interactions, we often decide who people appear to be before we give them a chance to show us who they are. We take the superficial cues and fill in the blanks to round out our stories. Based on our previous experiences, we often carry forth some level of bias.

Type of clothing: Is it clean? Tattered? Expensive?

Accent: Is it recognizable? Regional or international? Slight or heavy?

Race: What are the cultural stereotypes?

Level of attractiveness

Age: Is this person "too" young? "Too" old?

Physical ability: Can he or she manage without help?

While contextual cues are important and help to create a comprehensive picture, we have to be careful in maintaining enough objectivity to leave room for additional *factual* information.

With Mr. Smith, his physical limitations were obvious but many had made judgments about his cognitive abilities and capacity to cooperate. Some had decided his case would be a problem and didn't know how to address it, and others had pushed him aside figuring he didn't understand what was happening. Both scenarios are equally disturbing.

Seeing the Truth

If we are to deliver care to our patients, we have to be able to see them as they are-not as our scripted versions of who we believe them to be. We cannot afford for their needs to go unaddressed because we choose to stay loyal to our pre-constructed narrative. This is not care.

Recalling John Kabat Zinn's definition of mindfulness it began with,

> *"To purposefully pay attention in*
> *a sustained and non-judgmental way..."*

This is the practice of objectivity.

Never have I met a human being without bias. To ask that any of us constantly live in the space of objectivity is asking the impossible. However, to ask that we become more aware of our biases is crucial to the professional task at hand.

Chapter 11
NEEDS

We all have needs. The challenge comes in acknowledging those that are essential and how we are to address them. Further challenge comes in coordinating those needs with that of others.

Maslow's hierarchy of needs provides a solid framework through which we can evaluate areas being addressed or not.

This theory proposes that multiple levels of needs exist. It is often depicted as a five-level pyramid. Basic needs are represented near the bottom progressing to higher level needs near the top

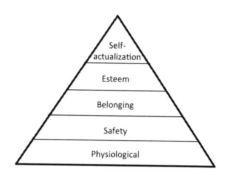

Many interpret this to mean that we generally require our lower levels to be met before we can place more focus on the higher ones.

In reality, multiple needs can be met simultaneously and different ones can dominate at different times. It's a complex dance in which we all knowingly and unknowingly engage.

The Bare Minimum

In the context of healthcare, needs are often pared down to a minimum. A patient comes to us for our services regarding an issue they have. We work to solve the issue and are rewarded with financial compensation.

This cold transactional script doesn't fare well for either party. When minimal needs are addressed, personal gratification remains elusive.

Patients may be left with a sense of disregard. This may in turn affect subsequent behavior regarding their health.

Did they feel comfortable enough to ask pertinent questions? Did they form a bond of trust with the practitioner? Were they made to feel a participant in their care? Will they choose to follow instructions?

As for the practitioners, they, too, may be lacking a sense of fulfillment. Did they rush the interaction to get through an impossible workload? Do they feel they are still contributing to the greater good or just collecting a paycheck?

This will impact overall satisfaction with their career and how they subsequently deliver care.

In each of their situations, a basic need was addressed (health problem and financial compensation) but emotional needs were left neglected. While every clinic, office or hospital operates differently, this very basic transaction has been at the core.

Innovative Approaches

Thankfully, there has been an emergence of more empathetic paradigms. For example, "dental spas" are intended to alleviate anxiety by incorporating relaxation services. A patient may be treated to reflexology prior to or during treatment.

There are interior designers who cater exclusively to medical offices. They transform the usual waiting room experience into something much more comfortable.

Taking this idea to the extreme is the Henry Ford West Bloomfield Hospital located in Michigan. The design and operations are like those of an upscale hotel.

Patients are considered guests who receive everything from wheelchair valets upon arrival to 24-hour room service. There's even an onsite greenhouse growing food that ends up on the restaurant -not cafeteria- menu.

The hospital boasts increased recovery rates and low readmissions.

Although most hospitals have a long way to go to reach this glorious standard, there is much that can be learned from the world of hospitality. The Ritz-Carlton Leadership Center brilliantly bridges the two realms.

They share valuable insight into enhancing the patient experience. Through their courses and advisory services, they show healthcare facilities how to incorporate their proven business practices to create more patient-centered environments.

As a result, their clients can expect more satisfied patients, better clinical outcomes, less mistakes, increased efficiency and improved employee engagement and retention.

There are those who would vehemently argue that patients are not hotel guests and do not come to hospitals for vacations. They argue that the trend towards "luxury" is at the expense of treatment.

While I do believe that hospitals are not the equivalent of resort facilities, there is no need to cling to outdated notions of what hospital stays should entail. Treatment outcomes do not have to decline because more patient needs are taken into account.

This is not about fancying up healthcare facilities. This is about creatively addressing aspects of patient care that have been long neglected. It is beyond my understanding why anyone would argue for the status quo when it clearly needs revision. If we truly value the populations we serve, we will strive to do better.

The bottom line is that patients tend to fare better when their emotional needs have been met in addition to the physiological ones. Furthermore, so do the healthcare workers that provide services to them.

Recalling Maslow's hierarchy, we have to cover more of the pyramid than just one basic element within in the bottom level. Everyone wants to feel seen, respected and valued.

If we are to create healthcare environments that encourage well-being for all involved, we must broaden our expectations. Shifting our focus from merely problem-solving to one that is needs-oriented is crucial.

Chapter 12
CONCLUSION

*"You are a human being
before you are a doctor."*

These were the words spoken to me by a very dear patient immediately after his procedure. He was expressing gratitude for our treatment of him while he was in our care.

Though we had just met that day, he unknowingly became the necessary catalyst for *Compassionate Competency* being written and published.

The truth is that I've wanted to share the ideas in this book for several years. However, I hesitated. I felt as if there were too many unanswered questions:

Is the content important enough?
Does it have relevance?
How will it be received?
What makes me an "authority?"

The Question of Importance

This wasn't a topic likely to come up in the usual professional circles. Traditionally, colleagues discuss things such as the latest innovations and treatments, new regulations, and marketing practices.

While those things are vitally important to one's professional success and ensure continued competence, they do not address the whole picture.

In those same circles, we're far less likely to discuss personal frustrations and lack of fulfillment within our careers. Indeed, it's often expected that we present with only the face of success and not much else.

Healthcare is unique. I strongly believe that in this field, we can no longer afford to ignore or downplay the critical roles we play, nor the personal toll it can take.

Health is a form of wealth. When patients show up in our clinics and hospitals, they entrust their greatest fortune to us.

If we are to attend to that fortune and provide the highest level of care possible, we must bring our full selves to each interaction. This level of presence is crucial for their sake and our own.

Patients come to us in vulnerability. The last thing they need is to be dealt with in a perfunctory manner. We must meet their needs with knowledge and expertise as well as compassion. In addition, we must give our own needs the same consideration.

Holding fast to this belief, I understood that this topic was important enough to not only be addressed but heralded.

The Questions of Relevance and Reception

The concerns I had about relevance and reception were nothing I could resolve intellectually. They could only be answered by testing the material in a public space.

In 2016, I submitted a proposal to the *American Dental Education Association* for their New Ideas sessions at their annual convention.

I worked furiously on my 20-minute presentation knowing I had to use a limited amount of time wisely. A couple of weeks prior to the event, I happened to glance at a Kripalu catalogue I received in the mail.

Curiously, I had never subscribed to the magazine. It had recently started to appear in my mailbox. In the center, was a featured article on Dr. Christina Pastan whom I mentioned in Chapter 7 regarding self-care.

I was compelled to reach out to Dr. Pastan after reading her story. It turned out that she, too, was scheduled to present at the ADEA convention.

Along with her colleague and a few students, they would share their findings on dental student stresses. They also would discuss the impact of the wellness initiatives introduced at Tufts University School of Dental Medicine.

At this point, I knew I was onto something. I understood that I was moving in the right direction. The timing couldn't have been more perfectly orchestrated.

Fast forward to the day of my presentation, I was slightly anxious leading up to the time. Although, I was confident the information would be useful to those who might be interested, I still wasn't sure what to expect.

Fifteen minutes before I was to present, a few people had gathered at the location. I silently told myself that if ten people attended, I would be satisfied although the space could hold much more.

After all, continuing education credits weren't offered for short sessions and several longer presentations were already in progress.

In the next fifteen minutes, the entire space was filled with some individuals standing. I estimate that approximately 75-100 people showed up to hear the topic of "Emotional Intelligence, Mindfulness and Tomorrow's Practitioner."

I no longer question the relevance of the topic or the interest level. The reception was phenomenal and the private discussions that ensued with members of the audience buoyed my beliefs.

It has become more than evident that we are hungry for more than what healthcare has offered in the past. This is in perfect step with today's patients expecting a different type of healthcare experience.

All parties are feeling the need for a revolution. *Compassionate Competency* aims to offer one aspect of that transformation.

The Question of Authority

The last concern I had in writing this book was questioning my right to do so. Surely there had to be more qualified individuals than me! Drowning in my own insecurities, I found myself altering the proposed structure of my work before I created a solid foundation.

I didn't believe that a book primarily based around my thoughts and observations could speak to an audience that leaned towards hard science. As a result, I found myself turning to traditional research and trying to build my work upon that.

Therein lies the irony.

In order to prove my competence and establish some sense of authority, I started using detached, traditional methods. Is this not what I was trying to address in the first place?

I was frustrated by how our humanity was not a central piece in the healthcare system; yet, I was putting aside the very human aspect of the message I wanted to deliver in favor of traditional ways.

The end result was stagnation.

It was impossible for me to write anything authentic when I was working from an indifferent perspective. Only when I reoriented myself to the heart of my message, was I able to bring a much stronger offering.

Reorienting itself to heart is what I believe 21st century healthcare must do.

The Heart of Healthcare

At the beginning of this book, I stated that for years I led a double life. I kept my personal quest separate from my professional one.

Surely, I showed empathy towards my patients and knew colleagues who did the same. However, there was little conversation, much less formal discussion, around the topic.

Most workplace environments operate in much the same way. They are devoid of self-examination outside of standard evaluation criteria. We're expected to keep the mushy stuff to ourselves.

I believe this is a major problem of society at large.

We tend to reserve what we call compassion for certain people in certain spaces. We see it as a practice we engage in with family and friends. We extend it in our households, our intimate communities, our volunteer work, and our places of worship.

Sometimes, we show compassion towards strangers but under specific circumstances-for example, a homeless person passed on the street.

But quite often, what we're practicing is not necessarily compassion. It may be pity. It could be condescension. Sometimes, it's self-interest.

A tangible bond to a person or to their story, is not a requirement. It is not something that we ration out on Sundays or when we volunteer for a cause. True compassion requires that we see the other regardless of who that other is.

Though all industries could benefit from an introduction of compassion on all levels, this is especially true for healthcare.

The definition of the word "care" is

> *"the provision of what is needed for the well-being or protection of a person or thing."*

As members of the healthcare community, we are charged with this responsibility. If we are truly invested in healing, we must treat patients at more than just the level of their physical condition.

This requires that we see through the eyes of our shared humanity. Through this lens, we remember that our patients are not cases to be solved. They are whole people.

We also remember that we are not scripted robots assigned to these cases. We can choose to lead with our humanity instead of solely with a professional identity. We, too, are whole people.

I echo the sentiment of my patient's words, "You are a human being before you are a doctor." It speaks on two levels.

He was speaking to me of my choice to lead with my humanity. His words were also a reminder that before any degree was conferred or license was granted, I was a human being. (I still am.)

Ultimately, no standard measure of competence can ever diminish that fact. Indeed, we need not continue operating in a system that does not take our humanness into account.

Whatever your role within the healthcare community, the care that you extend goes well beyond your clinical competence. Rest assured that an infusion of compassion into our professional spaces will transform everything for the better.

REFERENCES

1. Pink, D. H. (2012).*A Whole New Mind: Why Right-brainers Will Rule the Future*. New York: Riverhead Books.

2. Taylor, J. B. (2011).*My Stroke of Insight A Brain Scientists Personal Journey*. London: Hodder & Stoughton General Division.

3. Goleman, D. (1996).*Emotional intelligence*. New York: Bantam Books.

4. Ofri, D. M. (2018).*What Patients Say, What Doctors Hear*. S.I: Beacon.

5. Naghshineh, S., Hafler, J. P., Miller, A. R., Blanco, M. A., Lipsitz, S. R., Dubroff, R. P., ... Katz, J. T. (2008). Formal Art Observation Training Improves Medical Students' Visual Diagnostic Skills. *Journal of General Internal Medicine, 23*(7), 991–997.

6. (n.d.). Retrieved February 2017, from http://www.ihi.org/education/ihiopenschool/resources/Pages/MedicalStudentsTransferObservationSkillsFromPaintingToPatient.aspx

7. Dr. Terry Wahls: When Hope Returns [Audio blog interview]. (2017, April 24). Retrieved April, 2017, from http://www.goodlifeproject.com/dr-terry-wahls/

8. Goleman, D. (2011).*The Brain and Emotional intelligence: New insights*. Northampton, MA: More Than Sound.

9. Lofton, K. (2015, September 27). Trauma Workers Find Solace In A Pause That Honors Life After A Death. Retrieved August 14, 2017, from http://www.npr.org/sections/health-shots/2015/09/27/443104073/trauma-workers-find-solace-in-a-pause-that-honors-life-after-a-death

10. Carr, N. G. (2011).*The Shallows: How the Internet is Changing the Way We Think, Read and Remember*. London: Atlantic.

11. Medina, J. (2008).*Brain Rules: 12 Principles for Surviving and Thriving at Work, Home, and School*. Seattle, WA: Pear Press.

12. Makary MA, Daniel M. Medical error-the third leading cause of death in the US. BMJ. 2016;35

13. BJ Miller [Television series episode]. (2017, May 7). In*Super Soul Sunday*. OWN.

14. Shanafelt Tait D, et al. Changes in burnout and satisfaction with work-life balance in physicians and the general US working population between 2011 and 2014. Mayo Clinic Proceedings, 2015(90):12;1600–1613.

15. Kohn, L. T., Corrigan, J., & Donaldson, M. S. (2000). To err is human: Building a safer health system. Washington, DC: National Academy Press.

16. Brandt, B., PhD. (n.d.). Interprofessional Education and Collaborative Practice: Welcome to the "New" Forty-Year Old Field . Retrieved April, 2017, from https://nexusipe.org/informing/resource-center/interprofessional-education-and-collaborative-practice-welcome-new-forty

ADDITIONAL RESOURCES

Beckman H. B., Wendland M., Mooney C., Krasner M. S., Quill T. E., Suchman A. L., Epstein R. M. 2012. The impact of a program in mindful communication on primary care physicians. Academic Medicine, 87: 815-819.

Brondani M, Ramanula D, Pattanaporn K. Tackling Stress Management, Addiction, and Suicide Prevention in a Predoctoral Dental Curriculum. J Dent Educ. 2014 Sep;78(9):1286-93

Chen D, Lew R, Hershman W, Orlande J. A Cross-sectional Measurement of Medical Student Empathy. J Gen Intern Med. 2007 Oct; 22(10): 1434–1438.

Douglas HE, Raban MZ, Walter SR, Westbrook JI. Improving our understanding of multitasking in healthcare: Drawing together the cognitive psychology and healthcare literature. Applied Ergonomics. 2017;59, Part A:45-55.

Levinson W,Lesser CS,Epstein RM.Developing physician communication skills for patient-centered care. Health Aff (Millwood) 2010;**29**(7):1310–18.

Shapiro S.L., Astin J.A., Bishop S.R., Cordova M. (2005). Mindfulness-based stress reduction for health care professionals: Results from a randomized trial. International Journal of Stress Management, 12, 164–176.

Sherman JJ, Cramer A. Measurement of changes in empathy during dental school. J Dent Educ. 2005 Mar;69(3):338-45.

Rada, RE,, Johnson-Leong C. Stress, burnout, anxiety and depression among dentists. J Am Dent Assoc. 2004 Jun;135(6):788-94

Working Party of the Royal College of Physicians. (2005) Doctors In Society: Medical Professionalism in a Changing World: Report of a Working Party of the Royal College of Physicians. London: Royal College of Physicians.

Kabat-Zinn, Jon. *Wherever You Go, There You Are; Mindfulness Meditation in Everyday Life.* New York: Hyperion, 1994.

Center for Mindfulness
University of Massachusetts Medical School
www.umassmed.edu/cfm

Center for Mind-Body Medicine
Washington, DC
www.cmbm.org

ABOUT THE AUTHOR

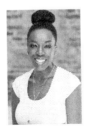

For over a decade, Dr. Frances Emelia Sam has been involved the realm of personal development and spirituality. Through her 360SOUL blog and speaking to various audiences, she has been able to share her message of moving towards compassion in personal and professional spaces.

Her work has been featured on several platforms including MindBodyGreen and the Huffington Post, which is also home to her Wise Women series. Contributors included Tara Brach, Byron Katie and Sharon Salzberg.

Dr. Sam is an Associate Professor of Oral and Maxillofacial Surgery at Howard University.

47162003R00080

Made in the USA
Middletown, DE
18 August 2017